HYPERTENSION DIET COOKBOOK

A Comprehensive Guide To Understanding Hypertension, Mastering Your Diet, And Living Well With Flavorful Recipes, Meal Plans, And Lifestyle Tips

Dr. Holmgren Alfred

DISCLAIMER

This book, "Hypertension Diet Cookbook" contains information that should only be used for informative purposes. It should not be used in place of expert medical advice, diagnosis, or treatment.

This book's material is derived from scholarly investigations, professional judgments, and the author's own experiences. Individual situations differ, though, so before making any dietary or lifestyle changes—especially if they have underlying medical issues like hypertension—readers should speak with a licensed healthcare provider.

This book's author disclaims all liability and responsibility for any outcomes that may arise from using the knowledge contained in it, whether directly or indirectly.

The author does not provide any express or implied warranties or representations regarding the completeness, accuracy, reliability, suitability, or availability of the content in this book, despite having taken every precaution to ensure its accuracy and reliability.

This book contains references and mentions of people, organizations, goods, websites, and other entities; these are merely for informational purposes and do not indicate endorsement. The only reason the stated entities are included is to give the reader more information or resources; the author has no financial or personal stake in any of them.

Before acting upon any advice or recommendations provided in this book, readers are urged to do their research and use good judgment.

Furthermore, dietary guidelines and recommendations could change depending on a person's tastes, allergies, and other health issues. Readers must adjust their diets to meet their unique demands and, if needed, seek professional advice.

By using this book, the reader accepts full responsibility for their actions and dietary and health-related decisions, and they acknowledge and agree to the conditions of this disclaimer.

ABOUT THIS BOOK

In the modern world of high speed and pressing health concerns, it is essential to know how to treat illnesses such as hypertension. The "Hypertension Diet Cookbook: Expert Guidance" is a priceless tool for anyone looking to improve their diet to take charge of their health.

This book is important not just for its thorough examination of hypertension but also for its useful advice on how to control it with diet.

Understanding the importance of diet is one of the fundamental tenets of treating hypertension. This book explores the role that nutrition plays in regulating blood pressure, highlighting the direct relationship between our health and the foods we eat.

By illuminating the connection between nutrition and high blood pressure, readers obtain important knowledge about designing a diet that promotes overall health.

This cookbook stands out for its useful advice on incorporating nutritional concepts into regular meals. The book gives readers the information and resources they need to make wise dietary decisions, covering everything from fundamentals like knowing portion sizes to more complex subjects like checking product labels for sodium content. It guides meal planning and preparation, enabling people to manage their diets sustainably.

The book's long lists of items to include and avoid in a diet that is friendly to high blood pressure are its main selling points. It gives users a recipe book for making balanced, tasty meals by emphasizing nutrient-dense foods including fruits, vegetables, whole grains, lean meats, and healthy fats. On the other hand, it assists readers in avoiding or limiting high-sodium, processed, and sugary foods, which can cause problems with their diet.

This cookbook's assortment of delectable and wholesome meals designed especially for those who are managing hypertension may be its most alluring feature.

There's something for every taste and occasion, from filling breakfast ideas to delectable lunch and dinner meals, as well as healthy snacks and decadent desserts. These dishes demonstrate that eating healthily can be both pleasurable and rewarding by placing equal emphasis on flavor and health.

In addition to recipes, the book includes useful resources including sample meal plans for various lengths of time and occasions, advice on dining out, and guidance during social gatherings.

A comprehensive approach to managing hypertension is provided by addressing lifestyle factors such as exercise, stress management, sleep, and at-home blood pressure monitoring.

"Hypertension Diet Cookbook: Expert Guidance" is essentially a full guide to leading a better life rather than just a cookbook. One delectable meal at a time, it enables readers to take charge of their health and well-being with its professional counsel, useful recommendations, and scrumptious recipes.

INTRODUCTION

The "Hypertension Diet Cookbook" introduction provides an overview of the main ideas covered in the book. It gives readers a general idea of what to expect and sets the stage for a discussion of dietary strategies for the management of hypertension. The author may discuss the global prevalence of hypertension in this section, emphasizing its importance as a significant public health concern.

The introduction may also discuss the possible side effects of unchecked hypertension, like renal damage, stroke, and cardiovascular disease. The introduction seeks to draw the reader in and highlight the significance of implementing dietary guidelines for successfully managing hypertension by framing the issue in this way.

Understanding Elevated Blood Pressure

The physiological factors that underlie hypertension are explored in detail in the section on understanding this condition.

It provides readers with a thorough explanation of hypertension, covering its description, causes, risk factors, and diagnostic standards.

The author may discuss how comorbidities, lifestyle decisions, and genetics affect the onset and course of hypertension in this section.

Additionally, the section may discuss the many forms of hypertension, clarifying their differences and therapeutic consequences, such as primary (essential) hypertension and secondary hypertension. This section gives readers a comprehensive overview of hypertension, enabling them to make educated decisions regarding their diet and overall health.

Diet Is Important For Managing High Blood Pressure

The significance of diet in controlling hypertension is a major topic covered in the "Hypertension Diet Cookbook." This section explores how dietary patterns affect blood pressure regulation, emphasizing the function of important nutrients, food groups, and dietary tactics in controlling hypertension. The DASH diet, which stresses the consumption of fruits, vegetables, whole grains, lean proteins, and low-fat dairy products while reducing salt, saturated fats, and added sugars, is one example of an evidence-based dietary plan that is introduced to readers. Additionally, the section might cover additional dietary components like potassium, magnesium, and alcohol consumption that affect blood pressure. This section equips readers to take proactive measures to improve their eating habits for better blood pressure control by clarifying the connection between diet and hypertension.

How This Cookbook Can Be Useful

The last section of the "Hypertension Diet Cookbook" describes how the book can be used as a useful tool for people who want to control their hypertension with diet. Here, the author might draw attention to some of the cookbook's standout qualities, such as its assortment of delectable recipes, adaptable meal plans, and useful lifestyle advice. The book informs readers about the different tools and resources available, such as cooking methods, meal preparation guides, and nutritional data.

The section might also highlight the cookbook's holistic approach, which combines dietary suggestions with lifestyle adjustments to support general well-being. This section intends to encourage readers to start their journey towards better health and hypertension management through knowledgeable food choices and culinary exploration by demonstrating the usefulness of the cookbook.

CHAPTER 1
BASICS OF HYPERTENSION AND NUTRITION

Elevated blood pressure in the arteries is the hallmark of hypertension, also referred to as high blood pressure, a chronic medical condition. Millions of people worldwide are impacted by it, and if left unchecked, there is a major risk of cardiovascular disease, stroke, and other consequences. Multiple blood pressure readings are usually necessary for the diagnosis of hypertension, which is divided into stages according to severity, from prehypertension to stage 2 hypertension. Recognizing the physiological mechanisms underlying hypertension is essential to comprehending its fundamentals. These mechanisms frequently entail problems in hormone control, increased blood volume, or vascular narrowing.

Nutrition is essential for the management of hypertension since food choices have a big impact on blood pressure.

There is a complex link between nutrition and hypertension that involves several dietary components, including fiber, salt, potassium, and magnesium. Furthermore, studies have shown that some dietary regimens, such as the DASH (Dietary Approaches to Stop Hypertension) diet, the Mediterranean diet, and plant-based diets, can effectively lower blood pressure and lower the risk of cardiovascular disease.

A thorough understanding of the fundamentals of nutrition and hypertension can help people adopt dietary practices that reduce the risks of high blood pressure and improve cardiovascular health in general.

A medical condition known as hypertension is defined by consistently high blood pressure values that are higher than usual. Two values are commonly used to measure blood pressure: the diastolic blood pressure, which indicates the pressure in the arteries between heartbeats, and the systolic blood pressure, which shows the pressure in the arteries during a heartbeat.

A blood pressure measurement within the normal range is 120/80 mmHg; readings that are continuously higher than this range are indicative of hypertension. Since the illness frequently shows no symptoms, it has earned the nickname "silent killer" because, if treatment is not received, it can gradually harm vital organs including the heart, kidneys, brain, and blood vessels, and create serious health problems.

Reasons And Danger Elements

A person's lifestyle, environment, and genetic makeup can all contribute to hypertension. The majority of instances of hypertension are primary, which develops gradually over time and is impacted by lifestyle factors like stress, physical activity, and food. Conversely, secondary hypertension is usually brought on by an underlying medical problem, such as obstructive sleep apnea, hormone imbalances, or kidney disease.

Many risk factors, such as age, family history, obesity, tobacco use, excessive alcohol use, high salt intake, and sedentary behavior, predispose people to hypertension. To effectively manage hypertension, preventive measures and early interventions must be put into place. This requires an understanding of these causes and risk factors.

Nutrition's Part in Controlling High Blood Pressure

The management of hypertension is significantly impacted by nutrition, as it has an impact on multiple physiological systems that control blood pressure.

Changes in diet can lower blood pressure, enhance vascular health, and lower the risk of cardiovascular events. Reducing sodium intake is one of the main nutritional strategies for managing hypertension since too much salt can cause fluid retention and an increase in blood volume, both of which can raise blood pressure. Foods high in potassium, such as fruits, vegetables, and legumes, help diuresis and vasodilation, which offset the effects of salt. Consuming meals high in fiber, calcium, and magnesium can also help maintain cardiovascular health and control blood pressure.

Crucial Elements For The Management Of Hypertension

Numerous important nutrients have specific impacts on blood pressure regulation and are crucial for managing hypertension.

For example, potassium lowers blood pressure by relaxing blood vessels and aiding in the maintenance of fluid balance.

Yogurt, bananas, oranges, potatoes, spinach, and other foods are high in potassium. Another essential vitamin that helps with blood pressure regulation is magnesium, which also promotes vascular health and muscle relaxation.

Leafy green vegetables, whole grains, nuts, and seeds are good dietary sources of magnesium.

Adequate consumption of calcium may assist in lowering blood pressure levels because it is necessary for nerve and muscle function as well as muscle contraction. Rich sources of calcium include dairy products, leafy greens, and fortified plant-based milk.

Moreover, fiber is essential for lowering blood sugar, enhancing lipid profiles, and inducing satiety—all of which help control hypertension. In a hypertensive diet plan, whole grains, fruits, vegetables, and legumes should be given priority as they are rich providers of dietary fiber. Focusing on these essential nutrients and embracing a well-balanced diet full of fruits, vegetables, lean meats, and whole grains can help people control their hypertension and lower their risk of heart problems.

CHAPTER 2
HYPERTENSION DIET PLANNING

Developing a well-organized diet plan is essential for the management of hypertension. This calls for a multidimensional strategy that takes into account several factors, including realistic goal-setting, knowledge of portion sizes, checking food labels for sodium levels, and the use of effective meal planning and preparation techniques. Setting realistic goals based on personal requirements and circumstances is essential to any hypertension diet plan's effectiveness.

To guarantee congruence with medical advice and individual health goals, these goals must be developed in concert with healthcare experts. Setting clear goals helps people monitor their progress and maintain motivation when following a diet.

Creating Reasonable Objectives:

A key component of successfully managing hypertension with diet modification is setting realistic goals. It entails taking a methodical approach to formulating realistic goals that complement one's food choices, way of life, and state of health.

These objectives could take many different forms, such as lowering sodium intake, controlling weight, consuming more nutrient-dense foods like fruits and vegetables, and following dietary recommendations like the Dietary Approaches to Stop Hypertension (DASH) diet. By setting specific, quantifiable goals, people can track their development, pinpoint areas for growth, and recognize their accomplishments as they go. Furthermore, establishing reasonable goals helps people feel empowered and self-sufficient, which empowers them to take control of their health and gradually modify their diet.

Comprehending Portion Sizes

Knowing portion sizes and how they affect blood pressure regulation and general health is essential to controlling hypertension with diet. To practice portion control, one must keep an eye on both the amount of food ingested and the nutritional value and sodium content of each dish.

The prevalence of enormous portions in today's food world makes this awareness more important, as they can lead to excessive calorie consumption, weight gain, and raised blood pressure. People can optimize their dietary habits to assist blood pressure management and general well-being by practicing mindful eating techniques and becoming familiar with suggested portion sizes for various food groups. Furthermore, employing visual signals to control portion sizes and encourage satiety without overindulging, such as using smaller plates and utensils, might be helpful.

Examining Food Labels To Determine Sodium Level:

The capacity to identify and restrict sources of sodium in the diet is critical for managing hypertension, as it is a major cause of high blood pressure. In this context, it is critical for people to read food labels since they help them spot hidden salt sources in packaged and processed foods and help them make educated grocery shopping decisions.

The sodium content per serving, the sodium percentage daily value (%DV), and the presence of high-sodium additives such sodium nitrate/nitrite and monosodium glutamate (MSG) are important details to check for on food labels. Furthermore, becoming familiar with words like sodium bicarbonate and sodium chloride which are frequently used to indicate sodium levels might help one read product labels more efficiently. People can minimize their sodium consumption and help control blood pressure by emphasizing low-sodium diets and including whole, minimally processed items in their diet.

Tips For Meal Planning And Preparation:

Keeping a tasty, healthy, and hypertension-friendly diet depends in large part on meal planning and preparation. To maximize nutrient intake and reduce sodium consumption, careful menu planning, food selection, and cooking techniques are required.

Developing balanced, varied menus that highlight whole grains, lean meats, fruits, vegetables, and heart-healthy fats while minimizing processed and high-sodium foods is a key component of a strategic meal-planning approach.

Cooking can be streamlined by batch cooking and prepping meals ahead of time, which will save time and energy during hectic workdays. Additionally, you can increase the flavor of food without using a lot of salt by experimenting with herbs, spices, and other flavor enhancers.

People can develop long-lasting eating habits that improve blood pressure control and general health outcomes by adopting these meal planning and preparation guidelines into their daily routines.

CHAPTER 3

FOODS TO INCLUDE IN YOUR HYPERTENSION DIET

Fruits and vegetables include a variety of vital nutrients and bioactive substances that are vital for controlling blood pressure, making them the cornerstones of a diet for hypertension. Rich in potassium, magnesium, fiber, and antioxidants, these naturally occurring foods are high in nutrients and have a major impact on blood pressure regulation and cardiovascular health. For instance, potassium lowers blood pressure via encouraging diuresis and vasodilation, which counteracts the effects of sodium, a major predictor of hypertension. Furthermore, fruits and vegetables' high fiber content aids in weight management and improves satiety, which may lower the risk of obesity-related hypertension.

A varied intake of vitamins, minerals, and phytochemicals is ensured by emphasizing a range of colorful alternatives; these nutrients are all linked to overall cardiovascular well-being.

Whole grains are an essential part of any diet focused on lowering blood pressure since they release energy slowly and support heart health in several ways. Whole grains have several health advantages because they contain all of the fiber, vitamins, minerals, and phytochemicals that refined grains lose during processing. Refined grains also lose their bran and germ layers. Whole grains, including oats, barley, and brown rice, include soluble fiber that has been linked to improved glycemic management and lowered blood cholesterol, two conditions that are linked to the onset and progression of hypertension. Additionally, eating whole grains has been associated with improved endothelial function and decreased inflammation, which supports the health of the arteries and the control of blood pressure. A diverse range of whole grain choices, such as bulgur, quinoa, and whole wheat products, can be included in the diet to assist in the treatment of hypertension and diversify the intake of nutrients.

Lean proteins, which are low in saturated fat and cholesterol and abundant in the essential amino acids needed for muscle maintenance, tissue repair, and overall physiological performance, are a vital part of a diet that is friendly to hypertension. Lean protein sources, such as fish, chicken, lentils, and tofu, reduce the risk of hypertension and cardiovascular disease more than fatty meats and processed meats. Omega-3 fatty acids are abundant in fish, especially fatty types like sardines, mackerel, and salmon.

These fatty acids have been shown to have anti-inflammatory and vasodilatory effects, which support cardiovascular health and blood pressure regulation. Legumes and tofu are examples of plant-based protein sources that also provide the further benefits of fiber, potassium, and phytochemicals, which help to further support the control of hypertension and general health.

When they are obtained from nutrient-dense foods like nuts, seeds, avocados, and olive oil and consumed in moderation, healthy fats are essential components of a diet focused on lowering blood pressure. These plant-based sources are rich in monounsaturated and polyunsaturated fats, which have been linked to better lipid profiles, decreased inflammation, and improved endothelial function—all of which support cardiovascular health and blood pressure regulation. Including omega-3 fatty acid sources such as walnuts, fatty fish, and flaxseeds can enhance the positive benefits on blood pressure and cardiovascular risk in general. To maximize the benefits of healthy fats for the cardiovascular system, it is crucial to regulate portion sizes and give priority to whole food sources of these fats while reducing calorie consumption and potential negative effects on lipid profiles.

Dairy products with low fat content can be incorporated into a well-balanced diet for hypertension, since they offer vital nutrients like calcium, vitamin D, and protein, without being overly high in saturated fat.

When consumed in moderation, low-fat dairy products like skim milk, yogurt, and cottage cheese can still provide significant nutritional advantages, even if some people prefer plant-based substitutes like soy or almond milk. Dairy products' high protein content helps with satiety and muscle maintenance, while calcium and vitamin D are essential for healthy bones and muscles.

Nonetheless, it is imperative to choose low-fat or fat-free types to reduce consumption of saturated fat, since it may have adverse effects on cholesterol levels and cardiovascular well-being.

In addition, people who have dietary preferences and limits related to dairy or lactose intolerance may want to look into substitute sources of these nutrients to guarantee sufficient consumption.

Herbs and spices are great complements to a diet targeted at hypertension since they improve flavor and palatability and have many health benefits. Numerous herbs and spices, including cinnamon, ginger, turmeric, and garlic, have long been utilized for their anti-inflammatory, antioxidant, and vasodilatory qualities in medicine.

Adding these aromatic herbs to food improves its flavor and helps control blood pressure and cardiovascular health in general. Garlic and ginger, for example, have been demonstrated to lower blood pressure and enhance lipid profiles; turmeric, on the other hand, has strong anti-inflammatory qualities that may help those with hypertension.

Additionally, utilizing herbs and spices to increase flavor lessens the requirement for excess salt and sodium, which are known to be factors in the development and aggravation of hypertension. Playing around with different herb and spice combos can help manage hypertension and promote general well-being while bringing excitement and diversity to meals.

CHAPTER 4
FOODS TO AVOID OR LIMIT

High-Sodium Foods: Consuming a lot of sodium can cause fluid retention and elevated blood pressure, which is a major cause of hypertension. Processed foods, canned soups, packaged snacks, and fast food products are among the foods that are rich in salt. Although the body needs very little salt to function properly, the abundance of processed and convenience foods in modern diets often results in excessive sodium intake. Excessive consumption of sodium can upset the body's electrolyte balance, especially the sodium-potassium equilibrium, which is vital for controlling blood pressure. It is recommended that people with hypertension consume less sodium to better control their condition.

This can be as simple as carefully reading product labels, selecting low-sodium substitutes, and preparing meals from scratch using fresh ingredients as opposed to relying on processed foods.

Foods that have been significantly modified from their natural condition by a variety of techniques, including cooking, freezing, canning, or packaging, are referred to as processed foods. High concentrations of sugar, bad fats, sodium, and other additives to improve flavor, texture, and shelf life are frequently found in these goods.

Packaged snacks, frozen dinners, deli meats, canned soups, and pre-packaged sauces are typical instances of processed foods. Because too much sodium can raise blood pressure, those with hypertension should be especially concerned about the high sodium content of processed meals. Furthermore, vital nutrients like vitamins, minerals, and fiber—all crucial for maintaining general health and controlling blood pressure—tend to be lacking in processed foods. Therefore, it is advised for those who want to improve their overall health and blood pressure control to consume fewer processed foods and instead choose entire, unprocessed alternatives.

Sugary Beverages: Drinking sugary drinks, such as energy drinks, soda, fruit juices, and sweetened teas, has been linked to several unfavorable health consequences, such as type 2 diabetes, obesity, and hypertension. These drinks usually have a lot of added sugar, which increases the risk of weight gain and insulin resistance, two conditions that lead to hypertension. Furthermore, sugar-filled drinks have little to no nutritional value and are empty calories, which increases calorie consumption without supplying necessary nutrients or satisfaction.

Frequent intake of sugar-filled drinks can also cause blood sugar levels to fluctuate, which can make hypertension and other cardiovascular risk factors worse.

For those looking to control their blood pressure and improve their general health, limit or stay away from sugar-filled beverages in favor of water, herbal teas, or unsweetened alternatives.

Red meat and processed meats: Saturated fats, cholesterol, and sodium, which are all linked to hypertension and cardiovascular disease, are frequently found in red meats like beef, hog, and lamb as well as processed meats like bacon, sausage, and deli meats.

Consuming large amounts of red and processed meats has been associated with a higher risk of hypertension and other illnesses like diabetes, obesity, and several types of cancer.

These meats' saturated fats have been linked to increased blood pressure and cardiovascular risk because they can increase LDL cholesterol levels and induce inflammation. Furthermore, processed meats frequently include additional chemicals and preservatives, which could hurt health. Thus, people can lower their blood pressure and enhance their general cardiovascular health by consuming less red and processed meat and opting for leaner protein sources like chicken, fish, lentils, and nuts.

Saturated and Trans Fats: Saturated fats are mostly present in meat, dairy, and egg products that come from animals, as well as in certain oils derived from plants, like coconut and palm oil.

Contrarily, trans fats are essentially synthetic fats made by hydrogenation, a procedure that solidifies liquid oils and lengthens the shelf life of processed goods. Research has demonstrated that fats, both trans and saturated, elevate low-density lipoprotein (LDL) levels and heighten the likelihood of cardiovascular ailments, such as hypertension.

These fats have the potential to cause atherosclerosis, a disorder marked by the accumulation of plaque in the arteries that can obstruct blood flow and raise blood pressure. Furthermore, the body may experience increased oxidative stress and inflammation as a result of saturated and trans fats, which could exacerbate hypertension and other cardiovascular risk factors.

Thus, cutting back on foods high in trans and saturated fats, like baked goods, fried foods, processed snacks, and fatty meat cuts, and switching to healthier fats like the mono- and polyunsaturated fats in nuts, seeds, avocados, and olive oil can help people control their blood pressure and lower their risk of heart disease.

CHAPTER 5

DELICIOUS HYPERTENSION-FRIENDLY RECIPES

Dietary interventions are extremely important in the current era of lifestyle disorders, especially when it comes to controlling problems like hypertension.

A hypertension-friendly diet is based on the idea of including foods and cooking techniques that support normal blood pressure levels. It places a focus on eating foods high in fiber, potassium, calcium, and magnesium and lowers cholesterol, saturated fats, and sodium intake.

To improve cardiovascular health, it also encourages including fruits, vegetables, whole grains, lean proteins, and healthy fats in a regular diet. Developing mouthwatering recipes that fit within a hypertension-friendly diet plan means choosing products and cooking methods carefully so that flavors are enhanced without nutritional value being sacrificed.

Ideas For Breakfast:

Breakfast is widely regarded as the most significant meal of the day since it determines an individual's energy levels and dietary intake. Breakfast ideas within the framework of a diet-friendly to high blood pressure concentrate on giving a healthy start to the day while taking into account dietary restrictions related to high blood pressure. Adding whole grains to morning foods, like quinoa, oats, or whole wheat bread, can provide a substantial and high-fiber base that encourages fullness and helps control blood pressure. Berries, bananas, and citrus fruits are examples of fruits that provide flavor and provide important antioxidants, vitamins, and minerals that are good for heart health. Lean protein sources like eggs, Greek yogurt, or tofu can also be added to breakfast dishes to improve their nutritional profile and maintain healthy muscle and metabolism. Innovative pairings of these components, such as oatmeal with nuts and fresh fruit on top or an omelet loaded with veggies, can turn everyday breakfast favorites into wholesome, delicious, and hypertension-friendly options.

Recipes For Lunch And Dinner:

There are plenty of opportunities to try out a wide variety of meals that are suitable for people with hypertension and suit varying dietary needs and tastes during lunch and dinner. To optimize nutrient consumption, these meals usually include a variety of fruits and vegetables in addition to a balance of proteins, fats, and carbohydrates. Whole grains that provide complex carbs and dietary fiber to support heart health and control blood sugar levels, such as brown rice, quinoa, or barley, can make a nutritious foundation for meals for lunch and dinner. To provide needed amino acids and control the amount of saturated fat, lean protein sources like fish, chicken, beans, or legumes can be added to main courses.

In the meanwhile, a range of vegetables—both cooked and raw—can enhance the meal's color, texture, and vital nutrients while also encouraging fullness and general well-being. You may improve the flavor of food without using a lot of salt or bad fats by adding aromatic herbs, spices, and healthy cooking oils like avocado or olive oil. People can satisfy their appetites and

follow the guidelines of a hypertension-
friendly diet while creating gratifying lunch
and dinner recipes by experimenting with
different cooking methods and ingredient
combinations.

Snacks & Starters:

Appetizers and snacks are important
components of the total dietary pattern
since they offer chances to sate appetites
and reduce hunger in between meals
without sacrificing overall health objectives.
It is crucial to choose nutrient-dense
snacks and appetizers that are low in salt,
saturated fats, and added sugars when
managing hypertension.

Fresh fruits and vegetables are great
options for guilt-free snacking since they
are low in calories and high in vitamins,
minerals, and antioxidants. They can be
eaten raw or combined with healthy dips

like hummus or Greek yogurt. Nuts and seeds are another healthy snack option since they provide heart-healthy fats, protein, and fiber that help with satiety and blood pressure control. If you're in the mood for something savory, air-popped popcorn seasoned with herbs or spices can fulfill your snack needs without adding too much salt or unhealthy ingredients. Similar to this, making whole grain crackers or muffins can fulfill your sweet tooth and help you reach your nutritional objectives.

People can enjoy a range of tasty snacks and appetizers that support a diet that is friendly to hypertension and overall well-being by being cautious of portion sizes and ingredient selections.

Sweets And Treats:

Desserts and treats are often associated with extra sugar and bad fats, so it may seem contradictory to include them in a diet that is friendly to hypertension.

However, it is still possible to prioritize cardiovascular health and enjoy sweet treats in moderation and with careful component selection. Making desserts at home gives you more control over the products you use.

You can use natural sweeteners instead of refined sugars, including honey, maple syrup, or fruit purees. Refined flour can be swapped out for whole grain flour and alternative flours like coconut flour or almond flour, which lower the glycemic impact of baked goods while increasing their fiber and nutritional content.

Furthermore, adding fruits to desserts—whether they be baked fruit crisps, compotes, or salads—adds natural sweetness and nutritional value without requiring the addition of added sugars.

While providing heart-healthy monounsaturated fats, experimenting with healthier fats like avocado or nut butter can also add to the richness and texture of desserts. People can indulge in sweet sweets that follow the guidelines of a hypertension-friendly diet by reinventing classic dessert recipes and adopting creative ingredient substitutions. This allows for occasional enjoyment without compromising long-term health goals.

CHAPTER 6
SAMPLE MEAL PLANS

Sample meal plans are organized dietary guidelines created to provide people with appropriate meals to assist them control their hypertension. These plans are usually designed to suit the dietary requirements and limits related to hypertension.

They specify meals and snacks for a week or two, for example. The main objective of the sample meal plans is to give people doable methods for implementing a healthy diet into their everyday routines, with a focus on lowering sodium consumption, boosting foods high in potassium, and enhancing cardiovascular health in general. These diets frequently incorporate a range of dietary groups, such as whole grains, fruits, vegetables, lean meats, and healthy fats, to guarantee sufficient nutritional intake and manage variables that lead to hypertension. People can improve their comprehension of portion sizes, food combinations, and meal timing—all crucial elements of a successful hypertension treatment strategy—by adhering to example meal plans.

Weekly Meal Plan

A one-week meal plan is a planned diet consisting of seven days that is intended to provide people with a thorough understanding of how to control their hypertension by eating a balanced diet. Breakfast, lunch, dinner, and snacks are usually included in this kind of meal plan, which emphasizes the inclusion of nutrient-dense meals that promote heart health and lower blood pressure. In addition to restricting salt, saturated fats, and added sugars, a well-designed one-week meal plan will frequently place an emphasis on the consumption of fruits, vegetables, whole grains, lean meats, and healthy fats.

People can create good eating habits, lessen their dependency on processed and high-sodium meals, and improve their control over blood pressure by adhering to a one-week meal plan. These meal plans can also be flexible and customizable to meet specific needs, dietary limitations, and cultural norms, which makes them an effective tool for encouraging long-term adherence to a heart-healthy lifestyle.

Weekly Meal Plan For Two Weeks

Like a one-week meal plan, a two-week meal plan helps people control their hypertension and improve their cardiovascular health by offering a planned dietary framework over a longer period—usually fourteen days.

By providing a wider range of food options and meal combinations, this extended meal planning strategy enables people to experiment with flavors, recipes, and cooking methods while still following the guidelines of a heart-healthy diet.

A thoughtfully designed two-week meal plan will include seasonal vegetables, a variety of protein sources, and healthy ingredients to provide both adequate nutrition and delicious food.

People can strengthen their healthy eating habits, lessen the monotony of meal preparation, and improve their capacity to maintain dietary improvements over time by extending the meal plan's duration to two weeks. A two-week meal plan can also help people plan their meals and grocery shop more effectively because they can stock up on necessary products in advance of their dietary requirements, which makes meal preparation more convenient and effective.

Organizing Meals For Special Events

Planning meals for special occasions entails modifying dietary plans and recipe ideas to fit festivities, vacations, or get-togethers while maintaining a focus on heart health and controlling high blood pressure.

This kind of meal planning acknowledges that people may find themselves in circumstances where their dietary objectives aren't aligned with traditional foods and culinary customs, but with careful preparation and inventiveness, it's still feasible to enjoy special events without jeopardizing cardiovascular health.

Planning meals for special events may entail lowering the amount of sodium in recipes, using healthier cooking techniques, and providing a range of nutrient-dense options to accommodate various dietary requirements and tastes.

Furthermore, people can also be proactive in informing hosts or event organizers about their dietary requirements to guarantee that appropriate meal alternatives are provided and to allay any worries regarding dietary restrictions. People can find a balance between indulging in celebratory foods and leading heart-healthy lives by including mindfulness and moderation in their meal planning for special occasions. This will ultimately promote general well-being and cardiovascular resilience.

CHAPTER 7
TIPS FOR DINING OUT AND SOCIAL EVENTS

Going out to eat and social gatherings pose particular difficulties for people trying to lead healthy lives, especially those with dietary restrictions like hypertension.

The temptation of decadent meals and the pressure from society to eat in groups can frequently result in overindulging in unhealthy foods that are heavy in sugar, fat, and sodium, all of which can worsen hypertension and other linked medical disorders. However, people can still successfully manage their blood pressure and stick to their nutritional objectives in these circumstances if they prepare ahead, practice mindfulness, and are aware of healthier options.

Those who have high blood pressure should choose their food from a menu carefully and strategically when dining out.

Choosing foods with reduced sodium, cholesterol, and saturated fats can help reduce the chance of making hypertension worse. Prioritizing meals with lean proteins, like grilled chicken or fish, as well as an abundance of veggies and nutritious grains, is one sensible tactic.

The nutritional profile of the meal can also be improved by asking for dish alterations, such as asking for dressings and sauces to be served on the side or changing high-sodium items to healthier ones.

A further important consideration is portion sizes since restaurant meals are usually greater than what is eaten at home.

People can enjoy eating out without going overboard by dividing entrees or choosing lesser servings.

Techniques For Events And Get-Togethers

Food is a major topic at parties and other social events, so it can be difficult for people with hypertension to go through these situations without giving in to unhealthy impulses.

However, these events can be enjoyed while still following dietary restrictions if they are planned and prepared carefully.

Eating a small, wholesome snack before the event can help control hunger and stop overindulging in bad foods. This is one helpful method.

Furthermore, staying on track with their dietary objectives can be facilitated by reviewing the available meal selections as soon as they arrive and giving priority to healthier options like fresh fruits and vegetables, lean proteins, and whole grains. Mindless snacking and the urge to overeat can be minimized by conversing and interacting with others away from the food table.

Last but not least, offering a meal that complies with dietary requirements helps guarantee that there is always at least one healthy option accessible and might even encourage others to make healthier decisions.

All things considered, managing eating out and social gatherings with hypertension necessitates a blend of awareness, planning, and calculated risk-taking.

People can enjoy these times without sacrificing their health or efficiently controlling their blood pressure by emphasizing nutrient-dense foods, choosing carefully from the menu, and paying attention to portion sizes. Furthermore, promoting healthier options and taking initiative can help create a welcoming atmosphere that promotes everyone's general well-being.

CHAPTER 8
LIFESTYLE TIPS FOR MANAGING HYPERTENSION

When it comes to managing hypertension, lifestyle changes are essential for lowering blood pressure and minimizing related health hazards. One of the most important of these changes is to exercise regularly.

It is impossible to exaggerate the significance of regular exercise in the treatment of hypertension. Regular exercise regimens are very important for preserving cardiovascular health and controlling blood pressure. Aerobic workouts that improve heart health, promote vasodilation, and improve vascular health, such as running, cycling, swimming, and brisk walking, have been shown to effectively lower blood pressure.

Exercises using weights or resistance bands that are part of resistance training can also help to develop muscles, which indirectly helps blood pressure control by increasing metabolic rate and encouraging weight reduction. Moreover, consistent exercise promotes the release of endorphins, which are neurotransmitters that lower stress and promote feelings of well-being. Stress is a major cause of hypertension.

Another important component of managing hypertension is learning stress management strategies because long-term stress can raise blood pressure and worsen cardiovascular risks. A range of strategies are included in effective stress management procedures to lower stressors and improve coping mechanisms. Cognitive-behavioral therapy (CBT), progressive muscle relaxation, deep breathing exercises, and mindfulness meditation are a few examples of these methods.

For example, mindfulness meditation focuses on accepting oneself without passing judgment and raising one's level of awareness in the present moment, which helps people develop more composure and calmness in the face of stress in life.

By triggering the body's parasympathetic nervous system, deep breathing techniques like diaphragmatic breathing or timed breathing promote relaxation and offset the physiological effects of stress on heart rate and blood pressure. Similarly, to relieve physical stress and encourage general relaxation, progressive muscle relaxation is methodically tensing and relaxing muscle groups. The integration of stress management approaches into everyday routines has the potential to cultivate resilience against stress and facilitate more consistent control of blood pressure.

Getting enough sleep is a crucial but sometimes disregarded aspect of managing hypertension. Sleep is essential for maintaining hormone balance, immune system function, and blood pressure regulation, among other physiological activities. Chronic sleep deprivation or poor-quality sleep has been linked to dysregulation of stress hormones like cortisol, disruption of circadian rhythms, and an elevated sympathetic nervous system, all of which can lead to cardiovascular dysfunction and high blood pressure. Therefore, for people with hypertension, it is critical to prioritize good sleep hygiene and use techniques to enhance the quality of their sleep. Better sleep quality and improved cardiovascular health can be achieved by following a regular sleep schedule, making sure your bedroom is free from distractions before bed, practicing relaxation techniques, and minimizing your exposure to stimulating activities just before bed.

Taking a blood pressure reading at home is a proactive measure that encourages people to take an active role in managing their hypertension. People who regularly monitor their blood pressure can see trends over time, see possible spikes or variations, and assess how well lifestyle changes and medication adherence are working.

A convenient and reliable way to take blood pressure outside of a clinical setting is with home blood pressure monitoring equipment, such as an ambulatory blood pressure monitor or a digital automated blood pressure monitor. People can work more productively with healthcare practitioners to customize treatment programs and make educated decisions about medication adjustments, lifestyle changes, and other interventions targeted at improving blood pressure control when they monitor their blood pressure at home. Additionally, home monitoring increases a person's sense of accountability and self-efficacy, enabling them to actively manage their hypertension and advance improved health outcomes.

CHAPTER 9
FAQS AND ADDITIONAL RESOURCES

Frequent Questions Regarding Diet And Hypertension:

Hypertension, also referred to as high blood pressure, is a global health issue that impacts millions of people. It is crucial to learn how to control hypertension with diet because it can have serious consequences like heart disease, stroke, and renal failure. This section tries to shed light and offer direction on often-asked topics about the connection between nutrition and hypertension.

A commonly asked question concerns the contribution of salt consumption to hypertension.

Table salt and processed meals are high in sodium, which has long been linked to high blood pressure.

As a result, people frequently ask about the appropriate daily salt intake and methods for cutting sodium without sacrificing the flavor of their food. Talking about the value of reading food labels, selecting fresh produce over processed foods, and enhancing flavor with herbs and spices are some ways to address this issue.

The effect of particular food patterns on blood pressure is an issue that is also often discussed. The DASH (Dietary Approaches to Stop Hypertension) diet, which emphasizes fruits, vegetables, whole grains, lean meats, and low-fat dairy while minimizing salt, cholesterol, and saturated fats, is a topic that people frequently ask questions about.

People can comprehend the potential advantages and viability of long-term adherence to the DASH diet by being informed about the scientific basis for the diet and its shown effectiveness in decreasing blood pressure.

A lot of people also want to know how drinking alcohol affects controlling their hypertension. While there may be some cardiovascular benefits to moderate alcohol consumption, excessive alcohol use can raise blood pressure and hasten the onset of hypertension. Giving advice on moderate alcohol intake, outlining typical drink quantities, and talking about substitute non-alcoholic options can help people make decisions that will support their blood pressure objectives.

Furthermore, concerns about the role that weight control plays in controlling hypertension are frequently raised.

The development and aggravation of hypertension are directly associated with excess body weight, especially abdominal obesity. It is crucial to clarify the significance of reaching and sustaining a healthy weight through a balanced diet and consistent exercise. Furthermore, dispelling myths regarding crash diets and encouraging long-term lifestyle changes for progressive weight loss can encourage people to take charge of their blood pressure control.

People also often ask for advice on how to handle social events and eat out while following a diet that is conducive to hypertension. Giving people helpful advice on how to order healthier food when dining out—like asking for dressings and sauces on the side, choosing grilled or steamed vegetables, and watching portion sizes—can help them stick to their diets without feeling deprived or alone in society.

Finally, concerns regarding the impact of lifestyle choices and stress management in the management of hypertension may surface. Chronic stress and unhealthy lifestyle choices, such as smoking, insufficient exercise, and poor sleep, can worsen hypertension and raise the risk of cardiovascular problems. To enhance the holistic management of hypertension, education regarding stress reduction techniques, the significance of regular physical exercise, the value of getting enough sleep, and resources for quitting smoking can be provided to individuals.

The "Hypertension Diet Cookbook" framework provides answers to frequently asked concerns regarding diet and hypertension, enabling users to make informed decisions and implement doable tactics to manage their blood pressure and enhance their general cardiovascular health.

Further Reading And Sources:

Apart from the extensive data included in the "Hypertension Diet Cookbook," those who are interested in receiving more guidance and assistance in controlling their hypertension with food may find several other useful sites. These resources, which provide a variety of viewpoints and insights about managing hypertension and good eating habits, come in a variety of media and include books, reliable websites, professional associations, and community support groups.

Books written by respectable medical experts in the fields of lifestyle medicine, nutrition, and hypertension are excellent resources for comprehensive knowledge and helpful advice. Books like "The Complete DASH Diet for Beginners" by Jennifer Koslo and "The DASH Diet Action Plan" by Marla Heller include meal plans, recipes, and step-by-step instructions designed to promote lowering blood pressure through dietary changes. These books are dependable resources for anyone navigating the challenges of managing their hypertension since they provide evidence-based recommendations based on scientific research.

Additionally, trustworthy websites run by academic institutions, medical associations, and government health agencies provide a plethora of trustworthy resources and information on dietary treatments and hypertension.

Websites like those run by the National Institutes of Health (NIH), the American Heart Association (AHA), and the Centers for Disease Control and Prevention (CDC) offer downloadable resources, educational materials, interactive tools, and evidence-based guidelines to help people make decisions about their lifestyle and nutrition.

Professional associations that focus on nutrition, hypertension treatment, and cardiovascular health are also essential for distributing important knowledge and encouraging community involvement. Membership-based associations like the American College of Cardiology (ACC), the American Society of Hypertension (ASH), and the Academy of Nutrition and Dietetics (AND) provide access to peer-reviewed journals, conferences, webinars, and educational events that highlight the most recent findings and clinical recommendations in dietary counseling and hypertension care.

Additionally, people can connect with peers going through similar struggles through online forums and community support groups, where they can exchange experiences, advice, and success stories regarding food and lifestyle changes for managing hypertension. Social media sites like MyFitnessPal, the r/hypertension forum on Reddit, and patient advocacy organizations like the American Heart Association's Support Network help people who are working to improve their cardiovascular health feel more connected to one another.

CONCLUSION

With tasty recipes, meal planning, and lifestyle advice, the "Hypertension Diet Cookbook" is a comprehensive resource for comprehending hypertension, mastering nutritional techniques, and leading a healthy lifestyle. Through answering frequently asked issues concerning nutrition and hypertension and offering more reading and resources, this cookbook enables people to adopt proactive measures for improved blood pressure management and cardiovascular health in general.

People can start along the path to better eating habits and ultimately improve their quality of life and lower their risk of complications connected to hypertension by receiving knowledge, support, and useful tools.